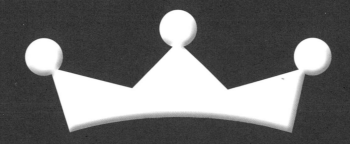

The Little King and his MARSHMALLOW KINGDOM

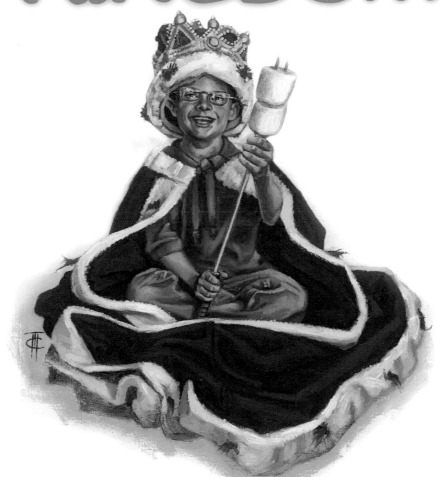

Louis Rotella III

Illustrated & Designed by Mark Chickinelli
Editorial Guidance by Tiffany Meyers

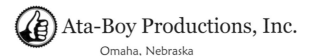 Ata-Boy Productions, Inc.

Omaha, Nebraska

ISBN 10: 0-9826842-1-5
ISBN 13: 978-0-9826842-1-4
Library of Congress Control Number: 2010903934
Cataloging in Publication Data on file with publisher.

Ata-Boy Productions, Inc.
c/o Concierge Marketing, Inc.
13518 L Street
Omaha, Nebraska 68137
www.MarshmallowKingdom.com

Editing: Tiffany Meyers
Layout and Design: Chickinelli Studios
Production and Marketing: Concierge Marketing, Inc.

Z 0102181   4/13

⌒

Printed in the United States
10 9 8 7 6 5 4 3 2 1

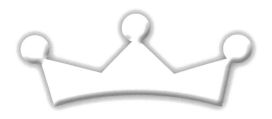

This book is dedicated to the three Lou's
who have shaped my life.

First, my grandfather, Louis Sr. His sense of integrity
is the standard against which every Lou since has
measured the strength of his own character.

Second, my father, Louis Jr., who treats everyone he
encounters with respect and regard—a quality that
separates the men from mice.

And then, of course, there's Louie the IV,
my wise (and funny) sage.

I love you, kiddo.

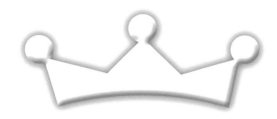

ACKNOWLEDGMENTS

This book would not have been possible if it weren't for a dream team of creative people.

Jill Rotella—my wonderful wife and partner-in-crime—was a wellspring of encouragement and ideas, not to mention a primary source for stories about the hilarity and tenderness that defines life with Louie.

Mark Chickinelli's ability to capture the essence of his subjects—from the expression in their eyes to the quality of their gestures—never ceases to amaze me. During his 30-year career, the extraordinarily gifted illustrator has worked with Fortune 500 companies and major advertising agencies across the U.S. Since 1981, he's produced our family bakery's advertising, but I've been lucky to call Mark my friend since childhood when he used to walk from his family's business to my family's business on a mission for baked goods.

Tiffany Meyers, a widely published writer and journalist, provided editorial guidance throughout. She underscored the importance of maintaining a sense of freewheeling fun in the text, not in spite of but because of, the complex themes in this book. She encouraged the use of language that respects our young readers' intelligence. I appreciate her heartfelt commitment to the book, which she once described to me as a "dream project."

I'm grateful to all of my friends and family—more people than I have room to list here—who reacted to this idea with genuine enthusiasm. It served to reinforce my own dedication to getting that final draft done.

Thank you, also, to the sweetest daughter ever, Mia, and the happiest of all baby boys, Niko, who teach me what matters in life.

Lastly, I'm forever indebted to my eldest son, Louis Rotella the IV. He's not just the inspiration for this book, but my whole life.

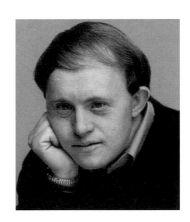

FOREWORD

The Little King, Louis IV, shows us what fun it can be to have an imagination and put it to good use in our everyday lives. He, like so many with Down Syndrome, brings such joy to his family, friends, and community. There is no doubt that those with Down Syndrome have put smiles on the faces of many.

It is my hope and desire that those with special needs will continue to create goals, strive to achieve those goals, and to never give up on their dreams. As I love to say, "It's our ability that matters most."

Here's to a great life with lots of marshmallows!

Chris Burke is best known for his TV role as "Corky Thacher" on the hit ABC show Life Goes On *and his recurring role as "Taylor," an angel, on the hit CBS-TV show* Touched by an Angel.

As an actor, singer, writer, and dedicated self-advocate, Chris has received numerous awards from local and national organizations for his tireless and inspiring work on behalf of people with disabilities. He has also been the Goodwill Ambassador to the National Down Syndrome Society and a Spokesperson for the National Down Syndrome Congress.

Chris Burke
"Corky"

—Chris Burke

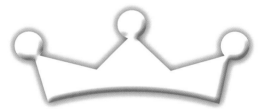

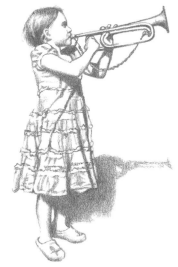

HEAR YE! HEAR YE! Let the trumpets blare!

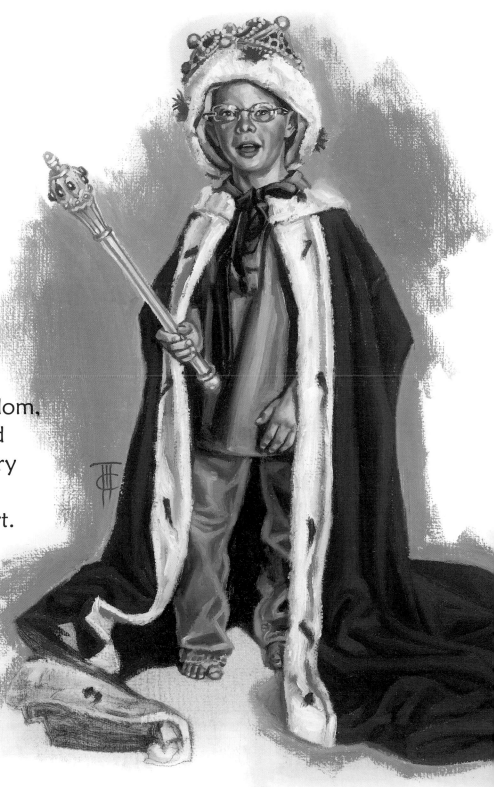

For I am King Louie.
King Louie the IV!
I rule over a place called
The Marshmallow Kingdom,
where it never rains, and
it never snows. And every
meal's a picnic—with
marshmallows for dessert.

YUM.

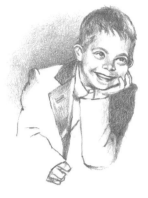

In my family—ahem, *excuse me!*
I meant to say:

In my *kingdom*, three Louie's came
before me: My dad, grandpa—and my
great granddad, too.

They're *all* named Louie, from one
to three. And then there's me:
Louie the IV!

'Tis a very **king-like** name,
don't you think?
A royal name
indeed!

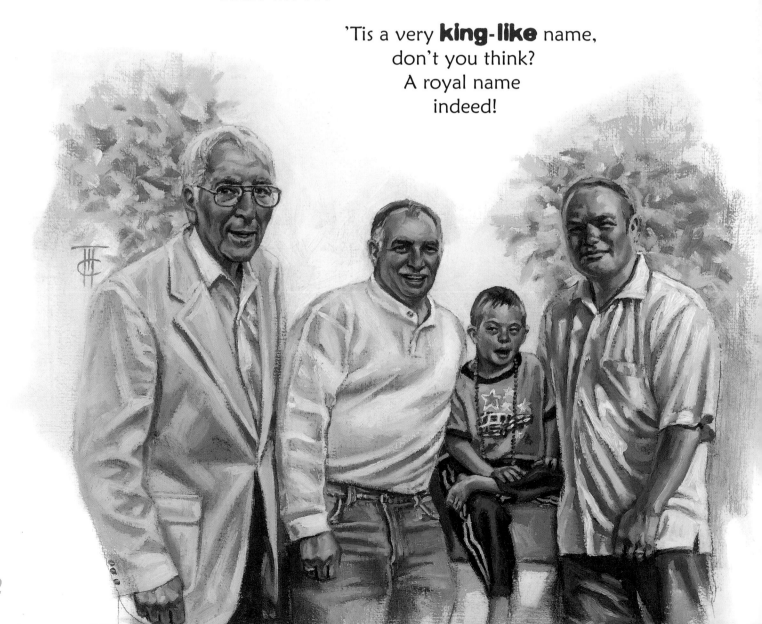

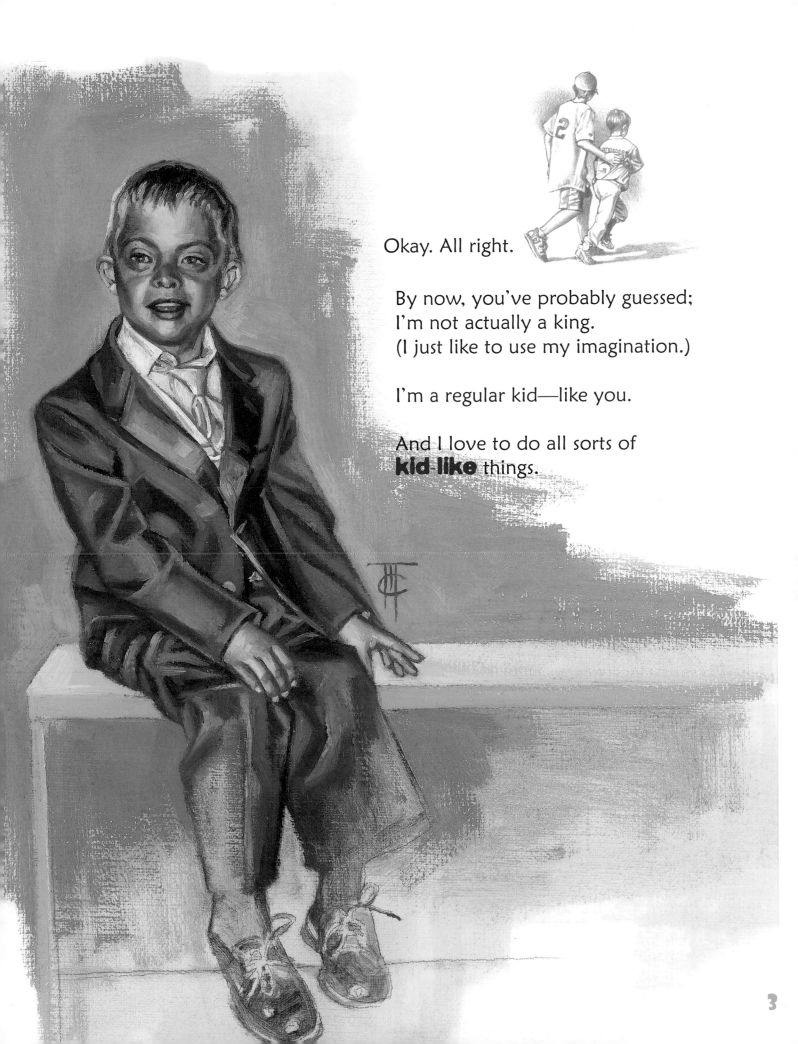

Okay. All right.

By now, you've probably guessed;
I'm not actually a king.
(I just like to use my imagination.)

I'm a regular kid—like you.

And I love to do all sorts of
kid-like things.

3

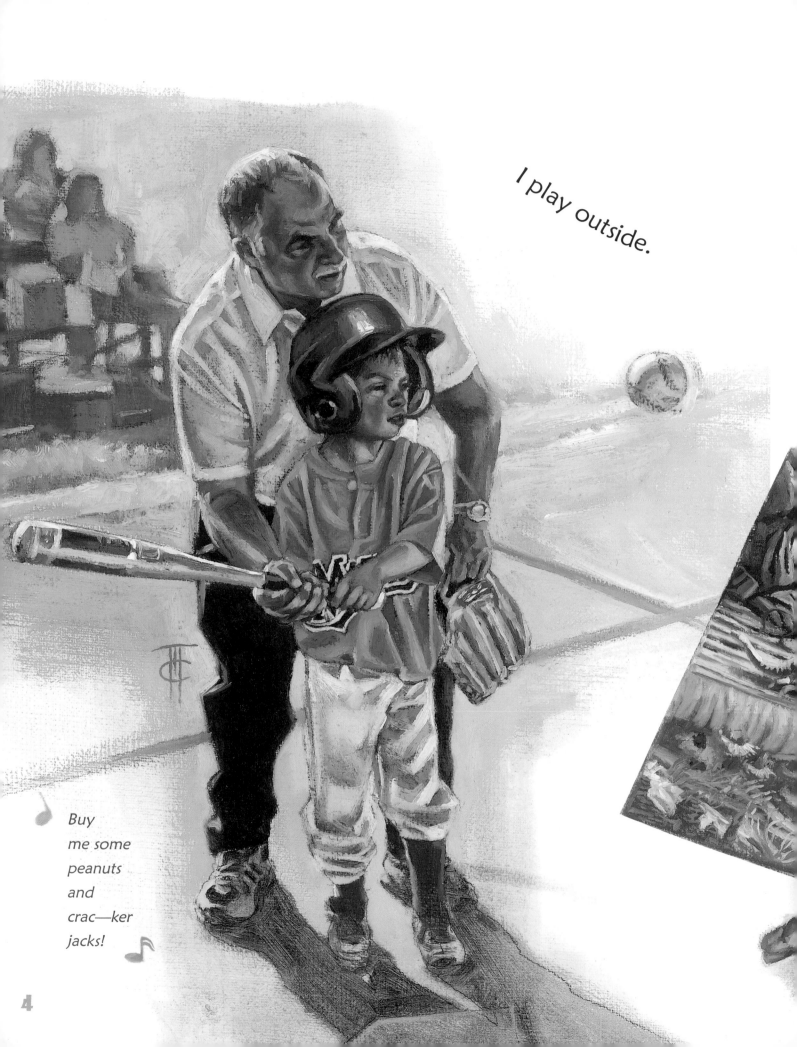

I play outside.

Buy
me some
peanuts
and
crac—ker
jacks!

4

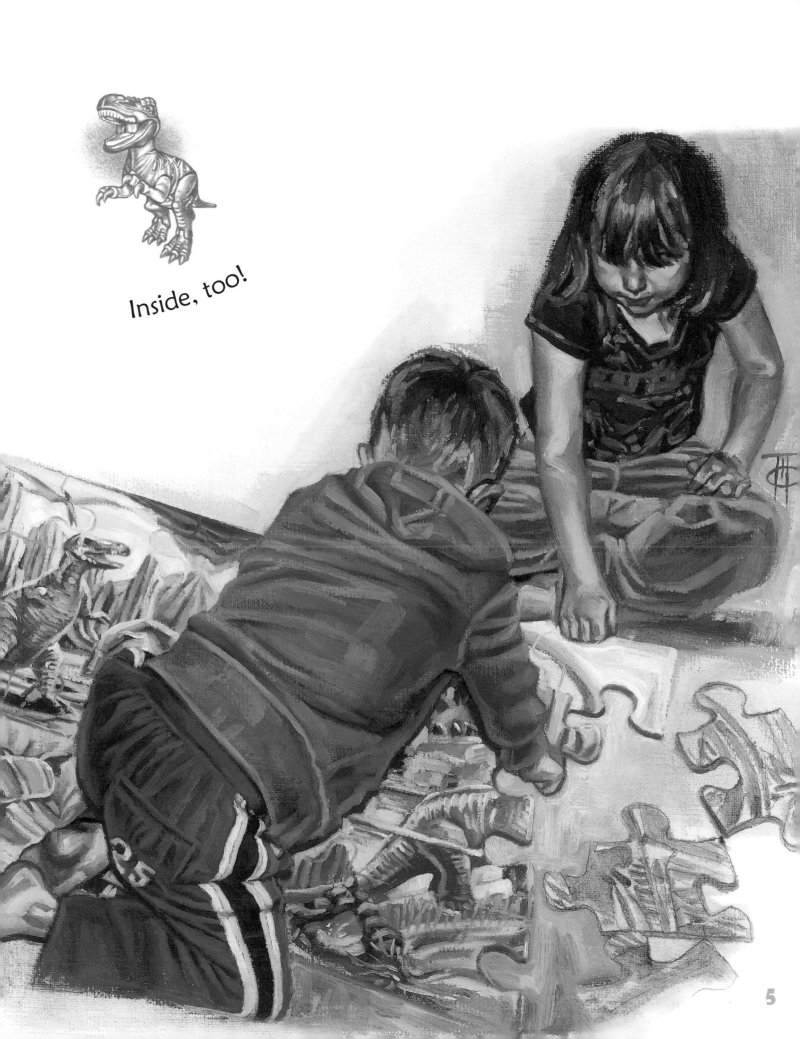

Inside, too!

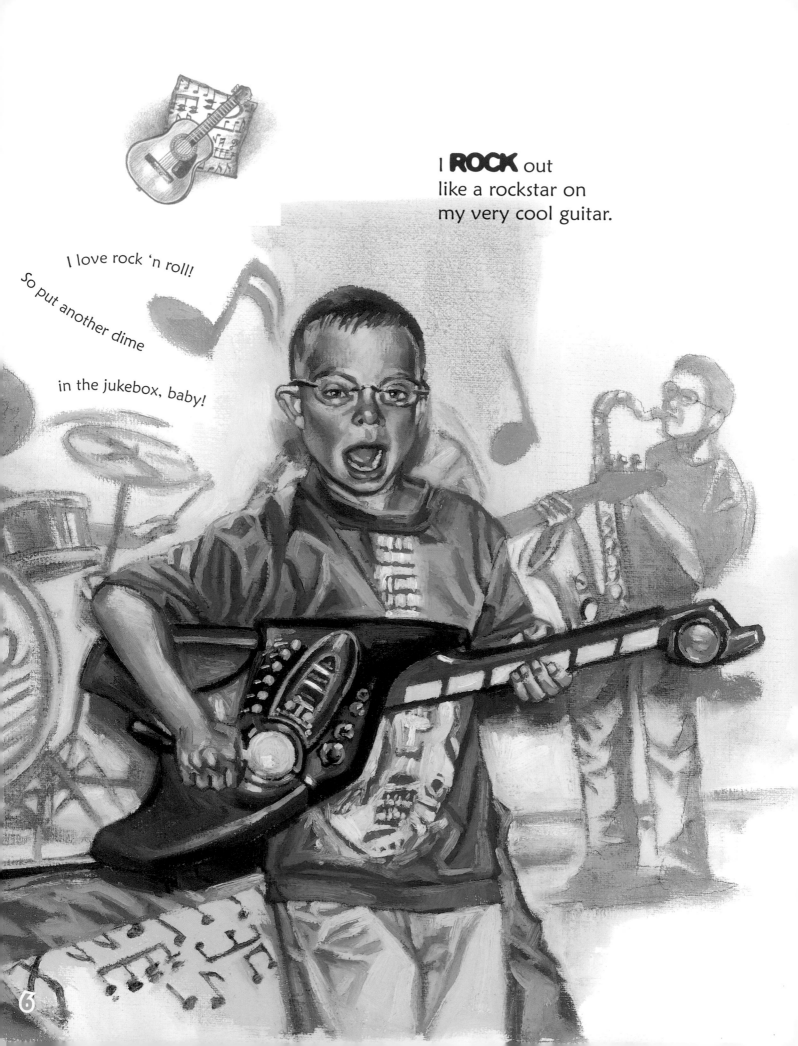

I **ROCK** out
like a rockstar on
my very cool guitar.

I love rock 'n roll!

So put another dime

in the jukebox, baby!

6

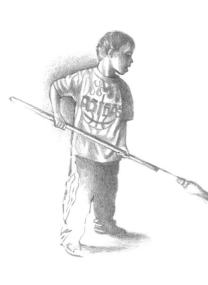

When grandpa Bill needs a hand,
I'm his man.

Just like he's always there for me.
(That's what families do.)

Oh, yes, indeed.
I'm a well-behaved fellow.

ALWAYS obedient.

PRACTICALLY perfect.

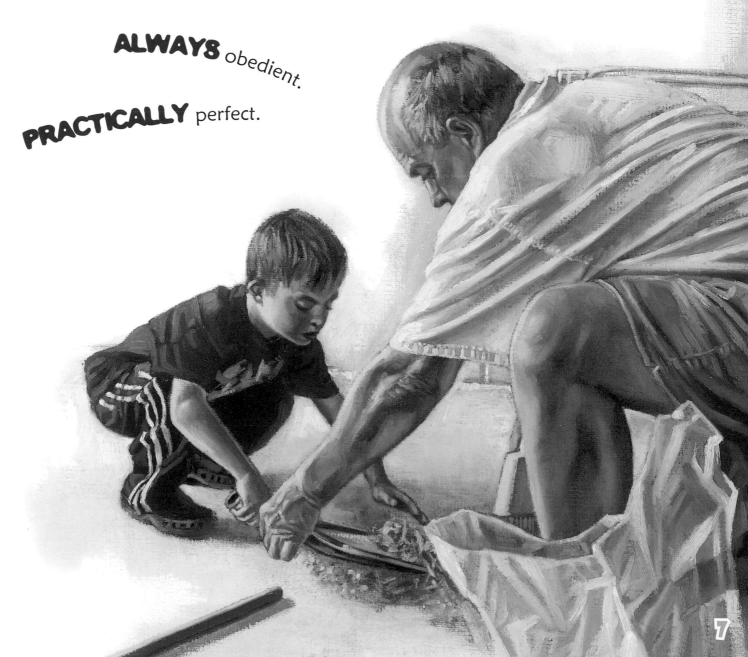

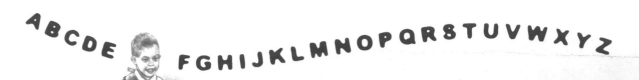

Okay. All right.

I'm sure you've guessed;
I'm not actually perfect.

In fact, from time to time,
I have been known to get into a little bit
(and really, I mean an itty bit) of mischief.

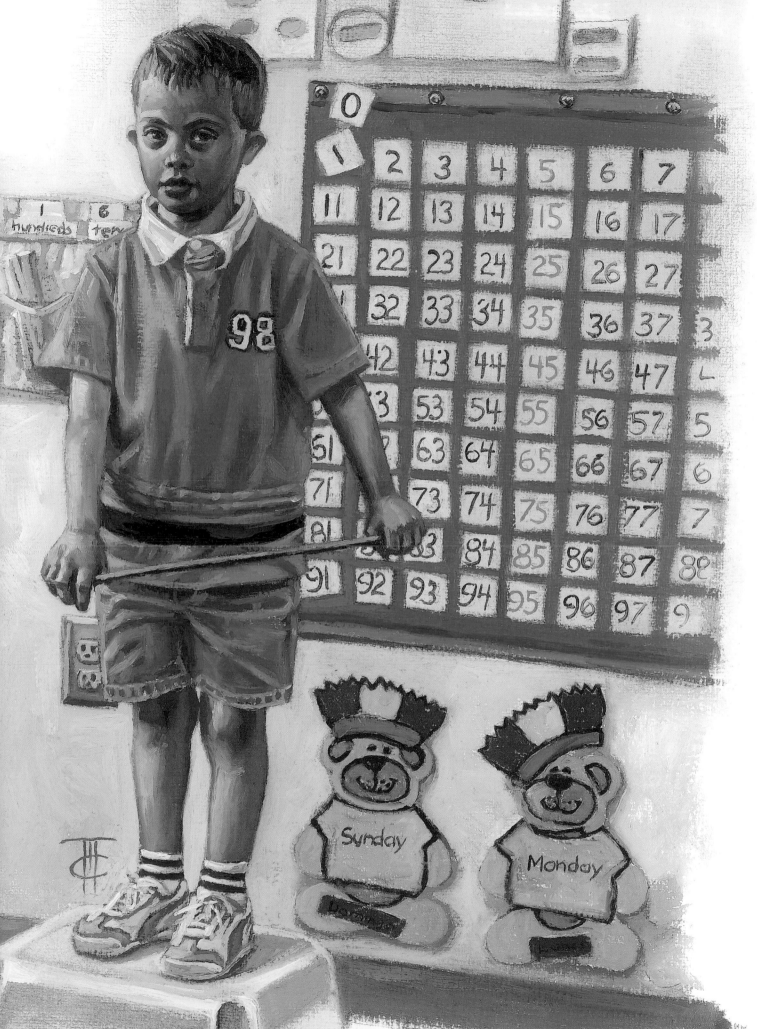

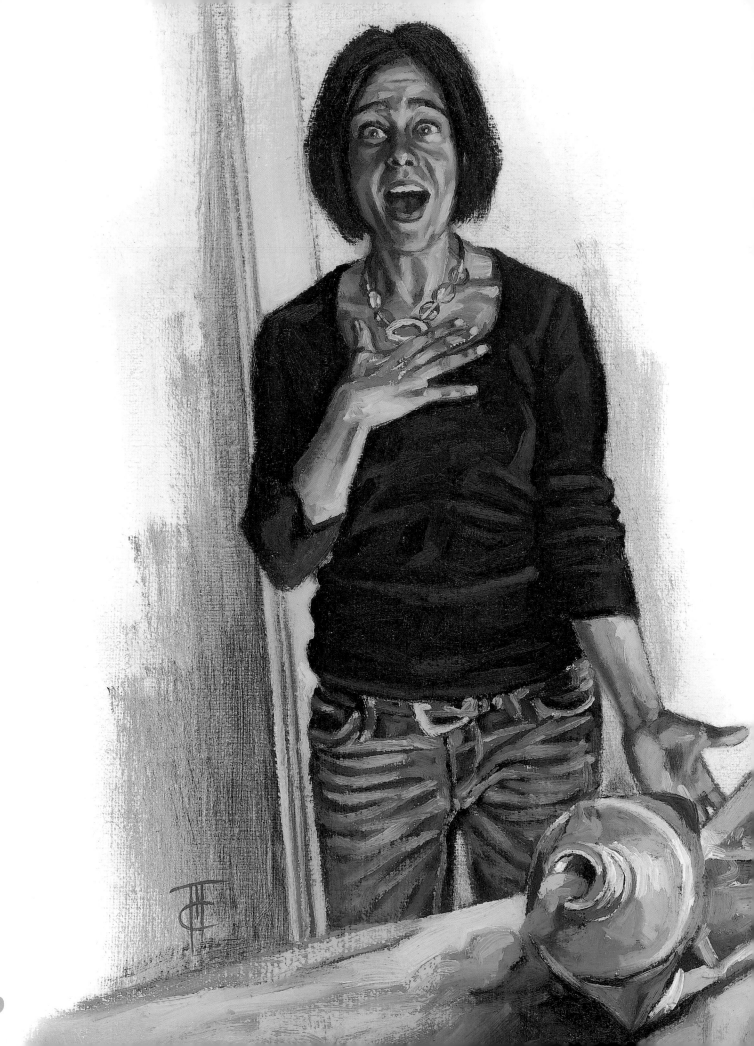

LOUIE! JOHN! ROTELLA! THE FOURTH!

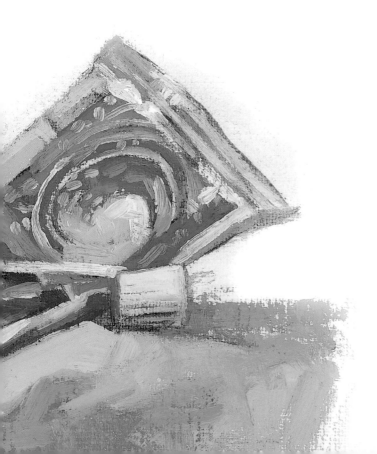

That's my mom, my darling mom, who was a teeny bit upset with me one morning.

Oh, but I couldn't resist. That tube of toothpaste was just sitting on a shelf.

I had to try it out...

...on my **HAIR!**

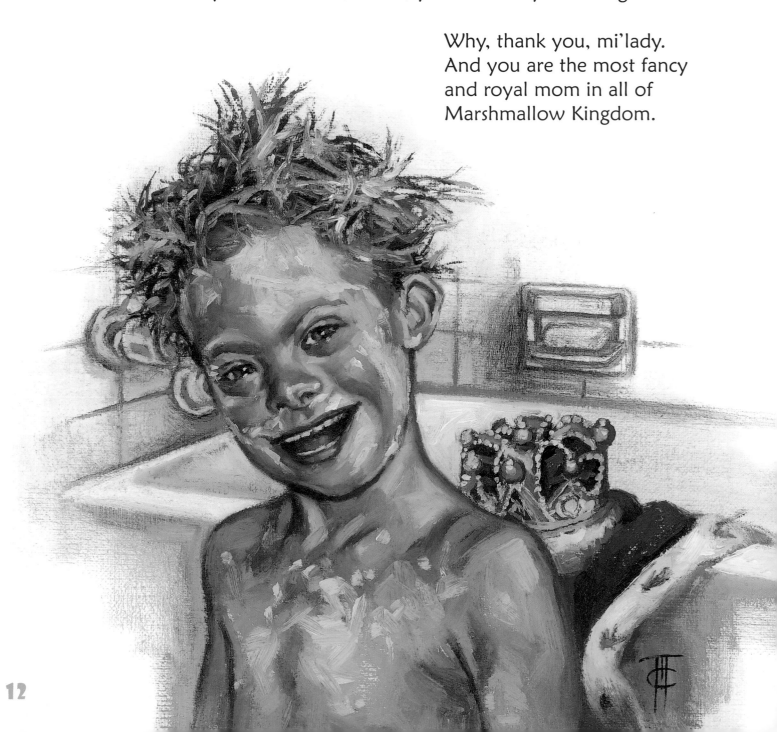

Mom called it "misbehaving." I called it a new hair-do.

But I noticed mom was trying hard not to laugh.
So I gave her a look, and that's all it took.

"Louie John Rotella, the IV," she said—only this time,
she was happy. She gave me a smooch. "Even when
you misbehave, buster, you're still my little king."

Why, thank you, mi'lady.
And you are the most fancy
and royal mom in all of
Marshmallow Kingdom.

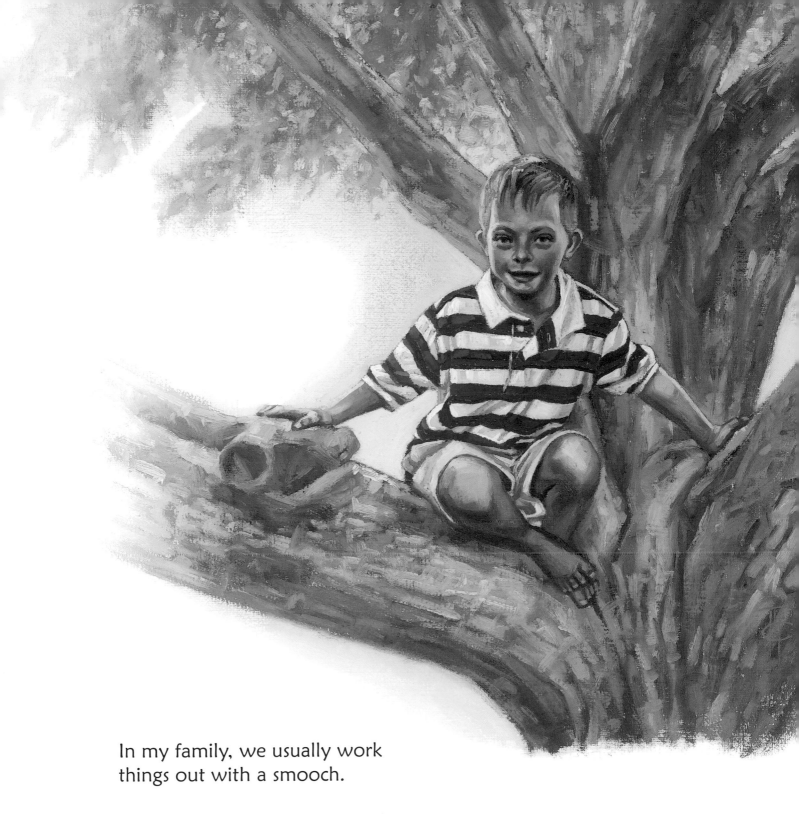

In my family, we usually work
things out with a smooch.

How about you? Do you ever get into mischief?
Just an itty bit of mischief?

Nobody's perfect, after all.
That's something we have in common.

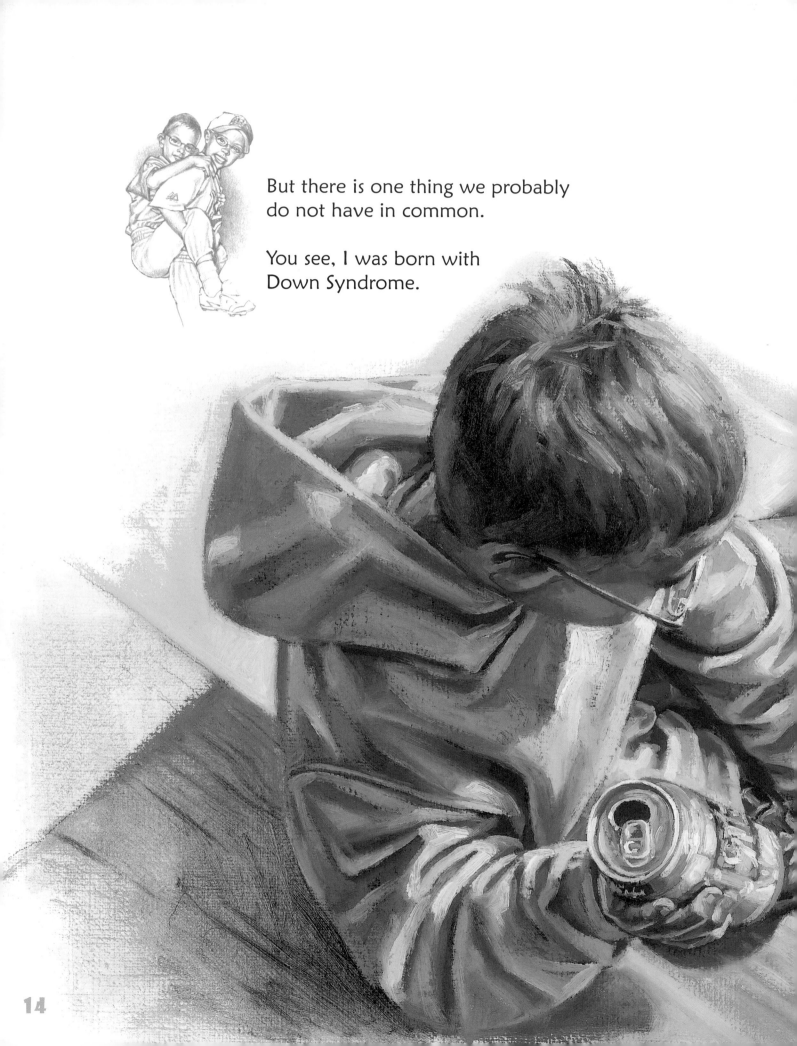

But there is one thing we probably
do not have in common.

You see, I was born with
Down Syndrome.

14

My buddy Shawn was also
born with Down Syndrome.
We don't talk about it much.
But that's because we just
understand each other.

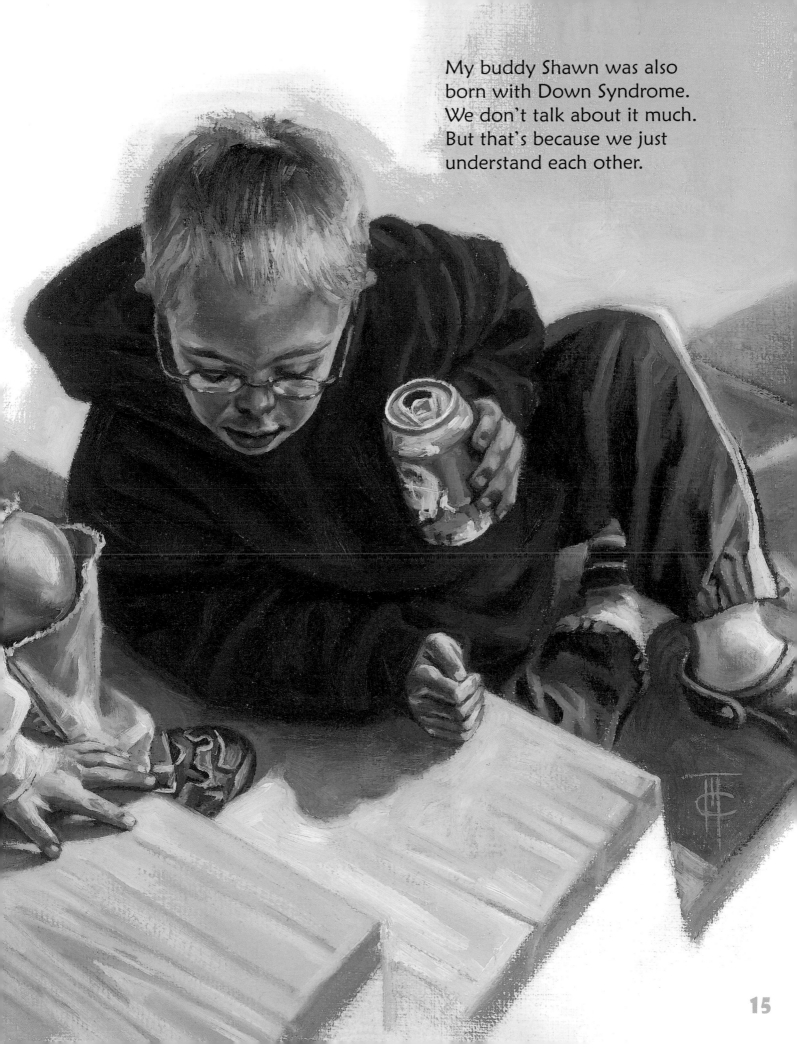

15

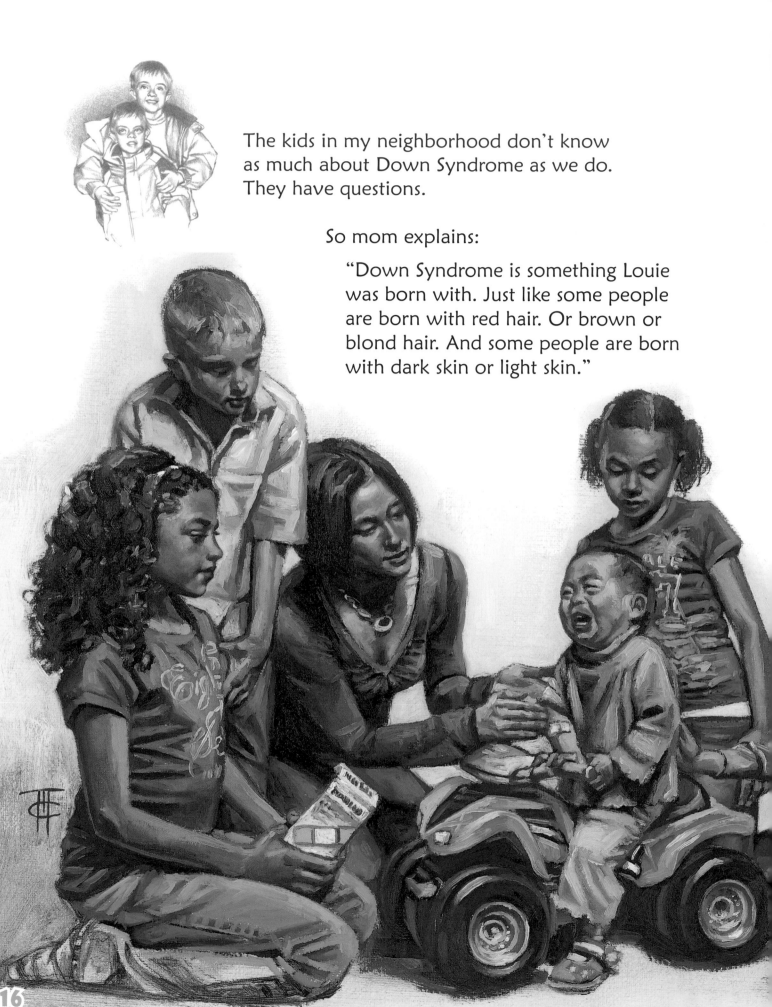

The kids in my neighborhood don't know as much about Down Syndrome as we do. They have questions.

So mom explains:

"Down Syndrome is something Louie was born with. Just like some people are born with red hair. Or brown or blond hair. And some people are born with dark skin or light skin."

"Or freckles!" says my cousin Taylor.

AHH-CHOO!

"Or allergies," says my other cuz, Kayla.

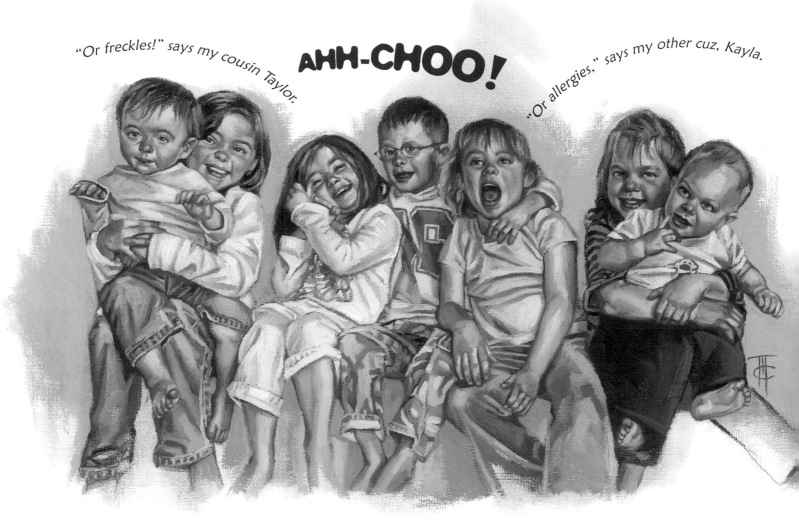

"Or the cutest giggle in
Marshmallow Kingdom,"
says Sara, gi*g*gling.
(Sara loves to use her imagination, too.)

My baby brother Niko has
other things on his mind.
If he could talk, he'd tell my sis:

"*MIA!* You're
SQUEEZING ME
too tight!"
(It's only because she loves him.)

"Freckles and allergies," says mom. "Exactly.
You were born with those things. They make
you different and unique. Down Syndrome
makes Louie different and unique. But in many
other ways, he's similar. After all, he's still a
kid—like you. Isn't he?"

17

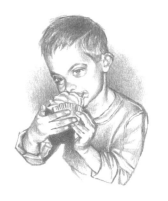

"Of course he is!" says Kennedy.
"And he loves to do **kid-like** things."

"Like have picnics with the
gang," says Mia. "With chicken
and carrot sticks—and marshmallows
for dessert."

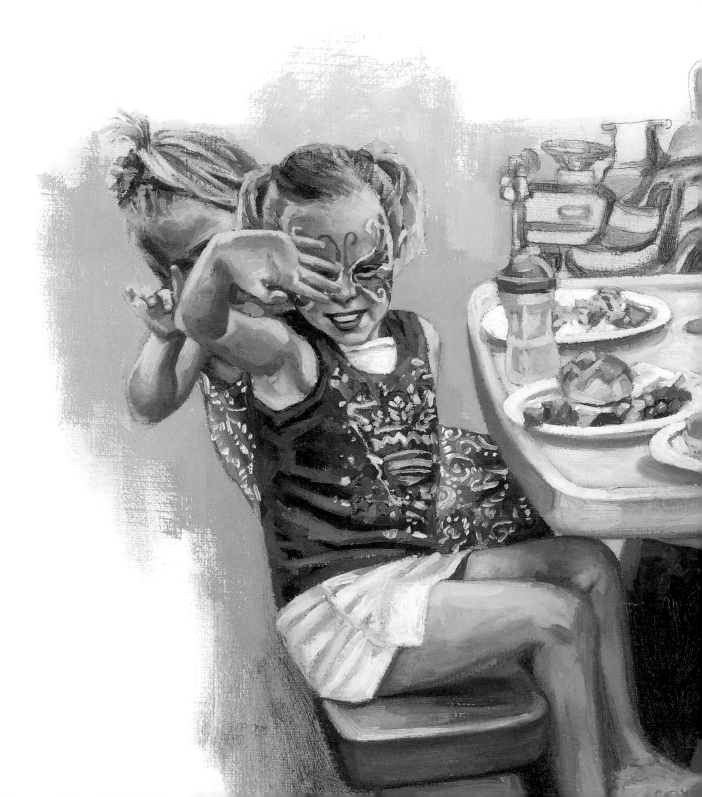

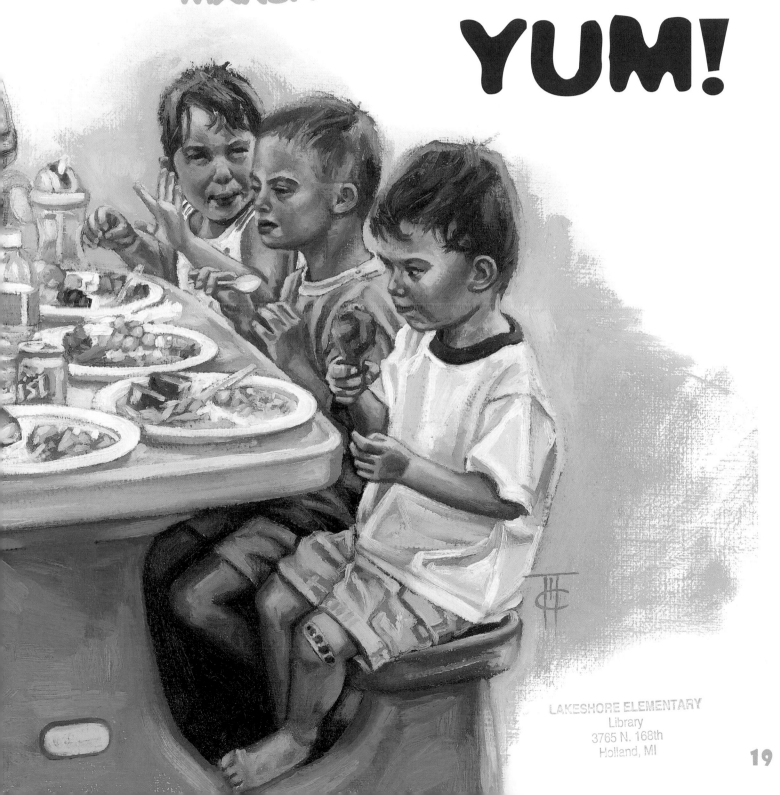

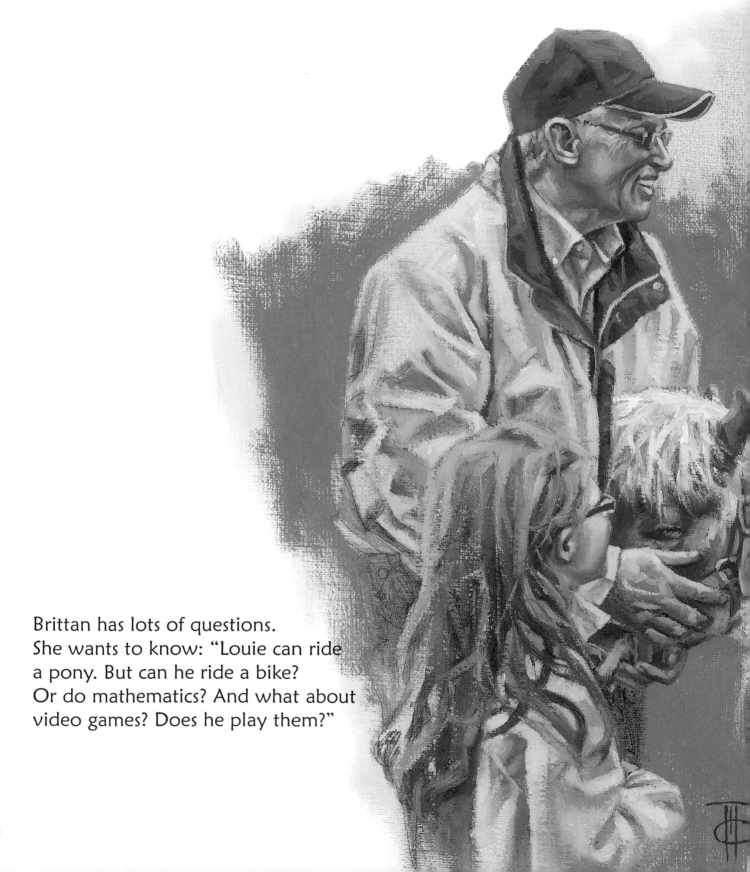

Brittan has lots of questions.
She wants to know: "Louie can ride
a pony. But can he ride a bike?
Or do mathematics? And what about
video games? Does he play them?"

Mom explains, "It might take Louie some extra time to do certain things. But if you give him a little help, you'll see that Louie can do lots of things."

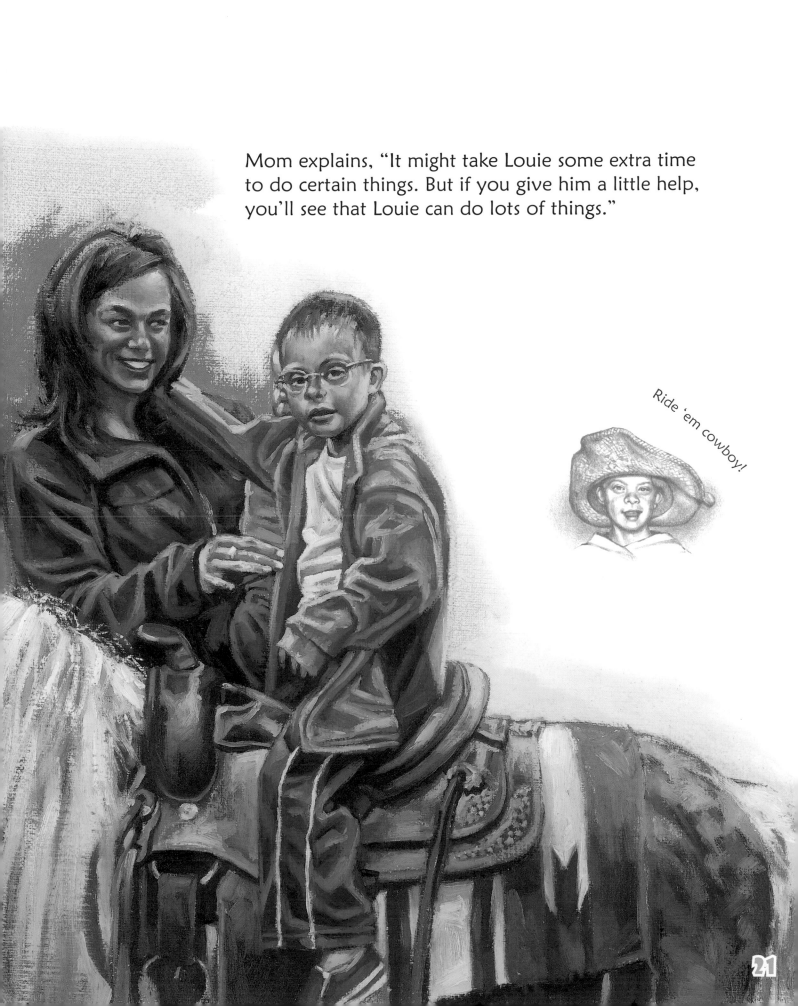

Ride 'em cowboy!

"Like bowl a **STRIKE!**" says Macie.

Macie's my very close friend. Even so, she doesn't know everything about me. She has a question. She wants to know...

"Can Louie go to the doctor and get a cure?"

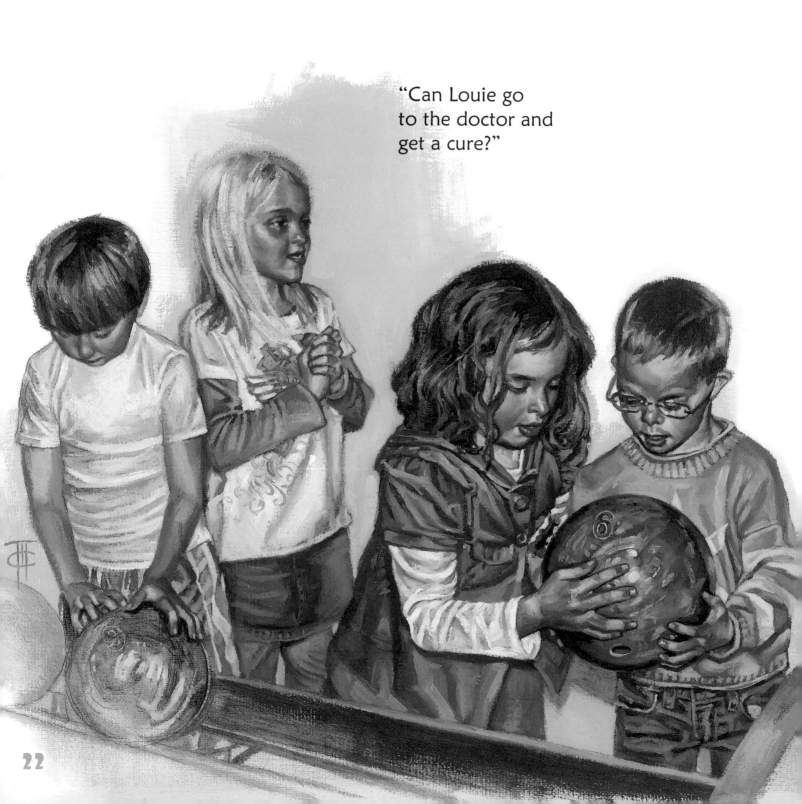

22

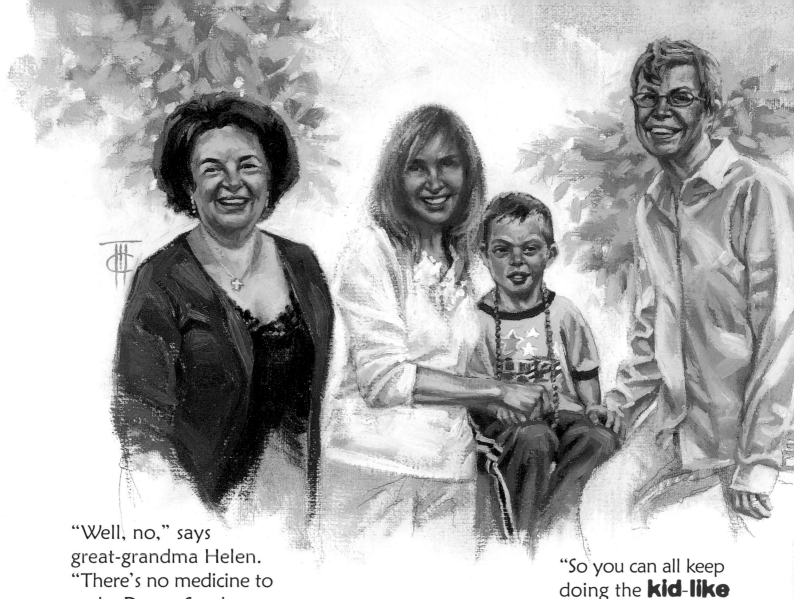

"Well, no," says great-grandma Helen. "There's no medicine to make Down Syndrome go away."

"But don't worry," says grandma Kathi. "You can't 'catch' Down Syndrome like you can 'catch' a cold."

"So you can all keep doing the **kid-like** things you love to do," says grandma Janet. "After all, you're all kids. Aren't you?"

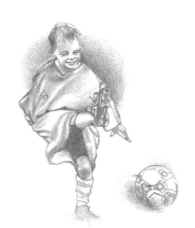

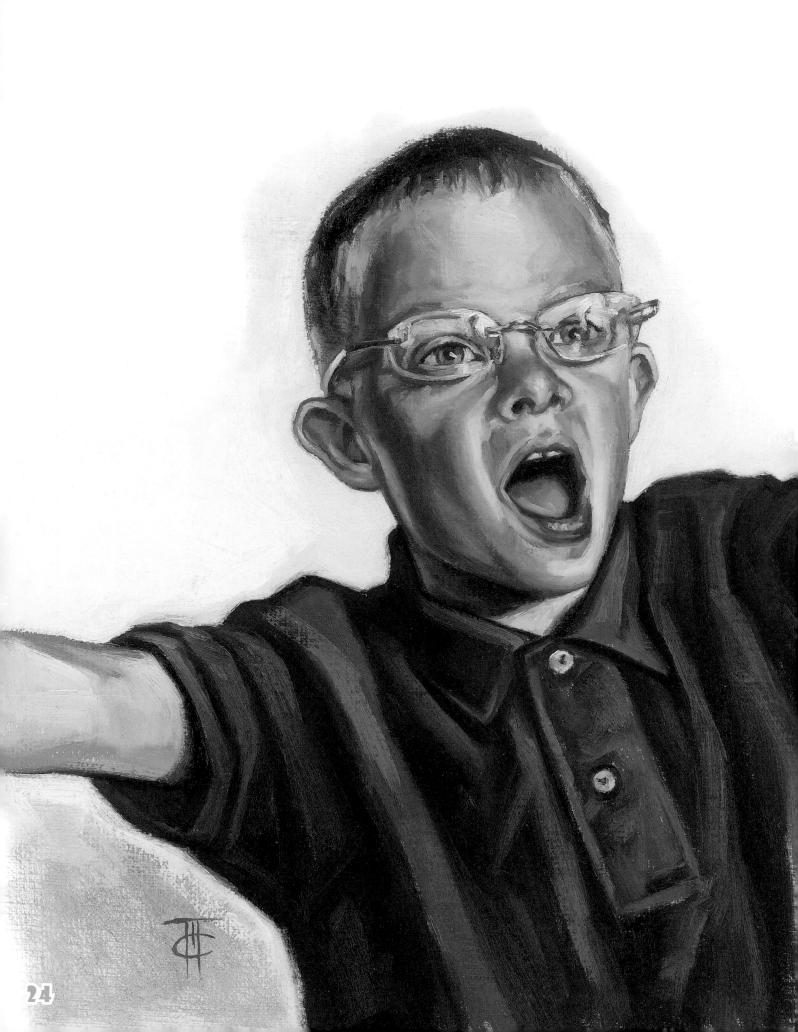

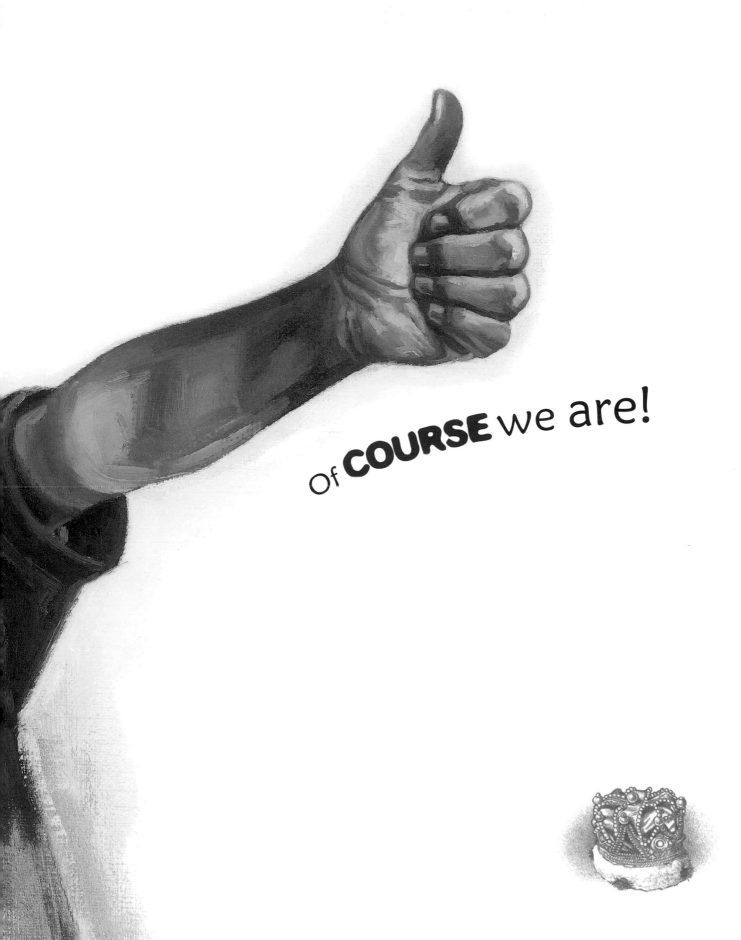

Of **COURSE** we are!

25

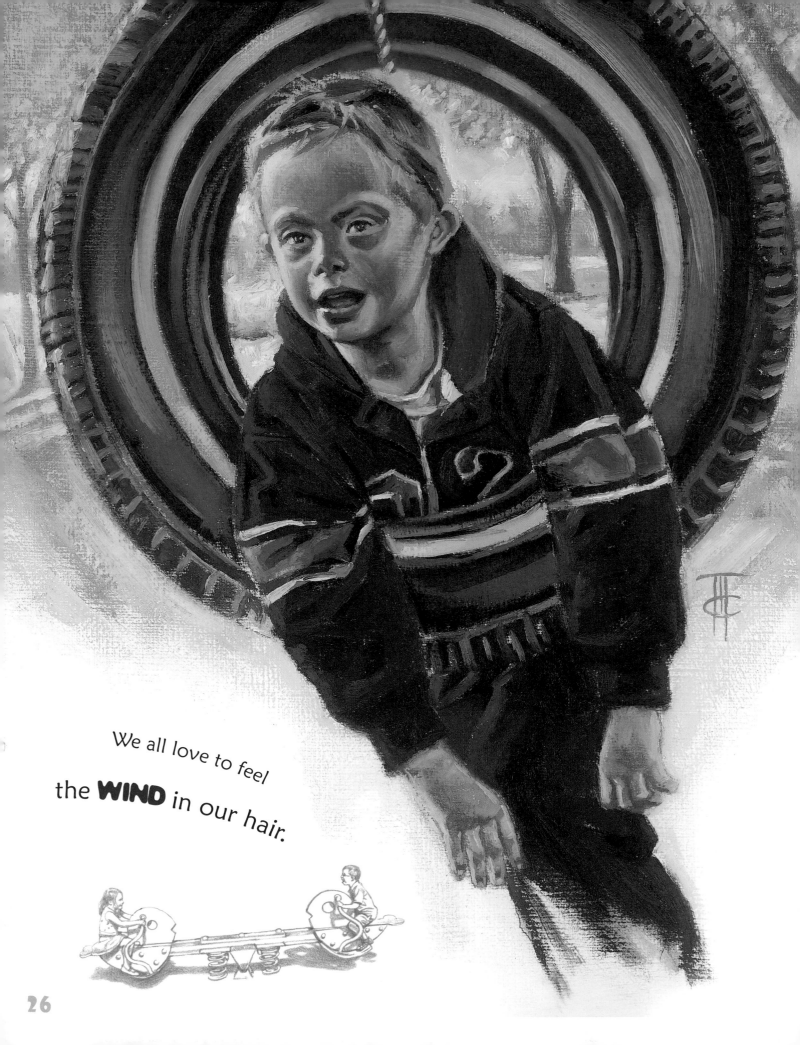

We all love to feel
the **WIND** in our hair.

26

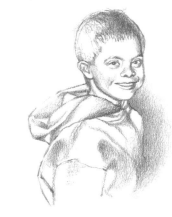

And to snuggle with furry little animals.

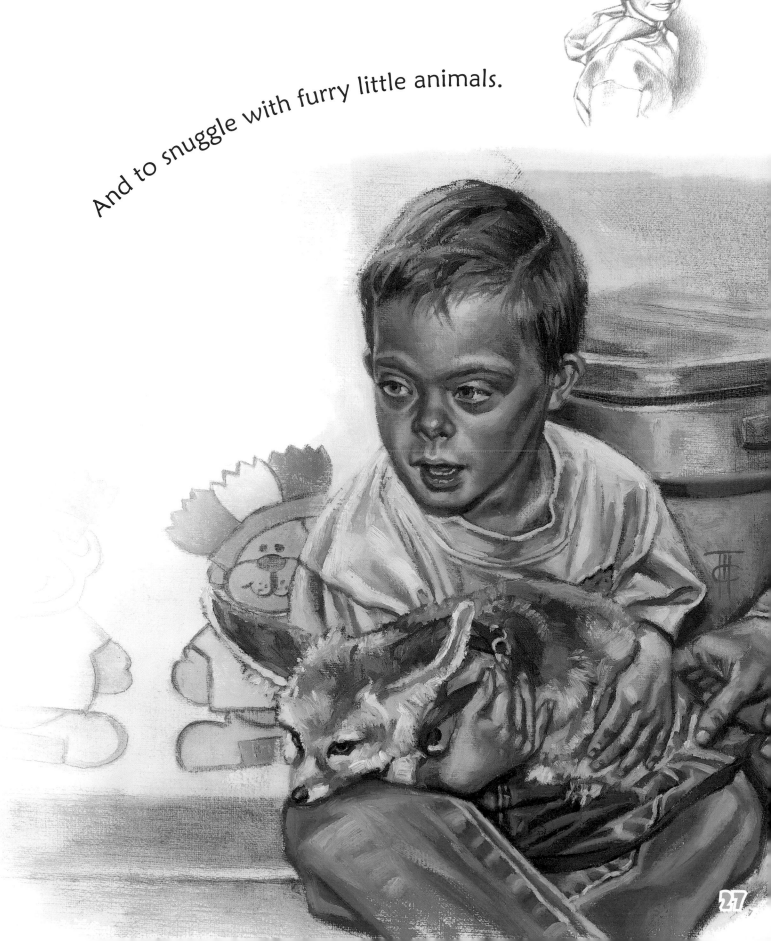

27

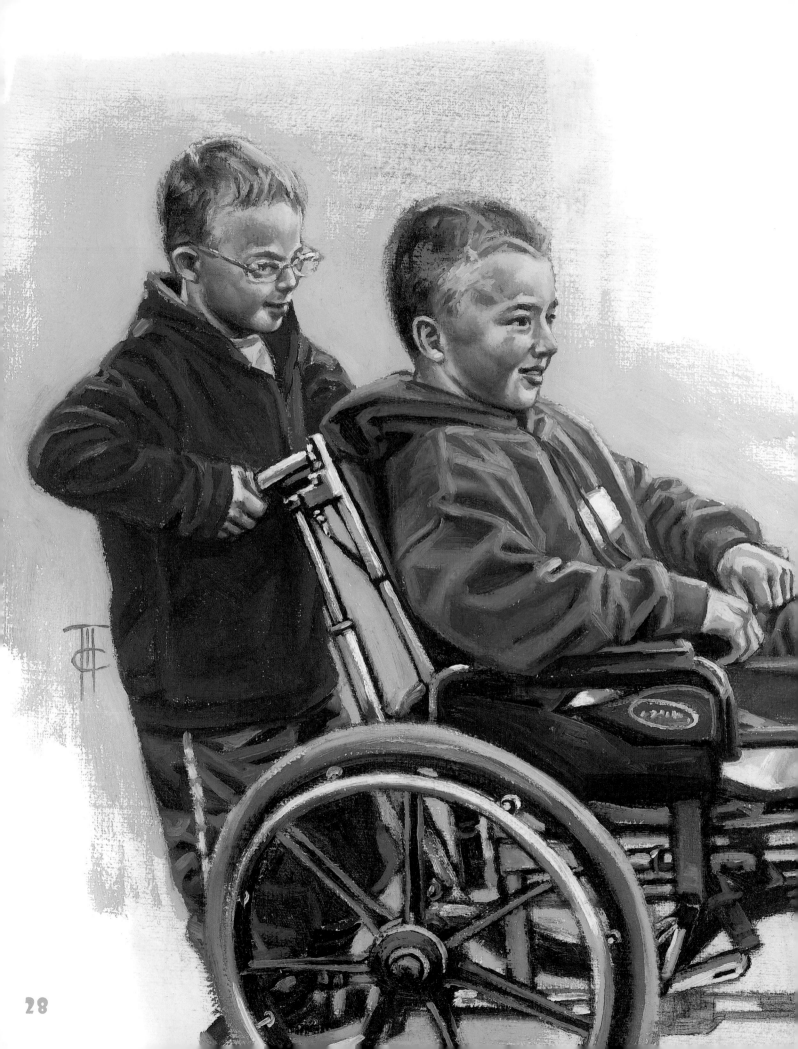

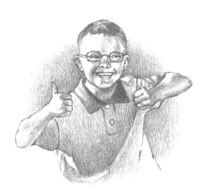

We love to help our friends,
like when Jared hurt his foot.

I helped him get around town,
because he would do the same for me.
(That's what friends do.)

Now, if only I could **POP** a wheelie!

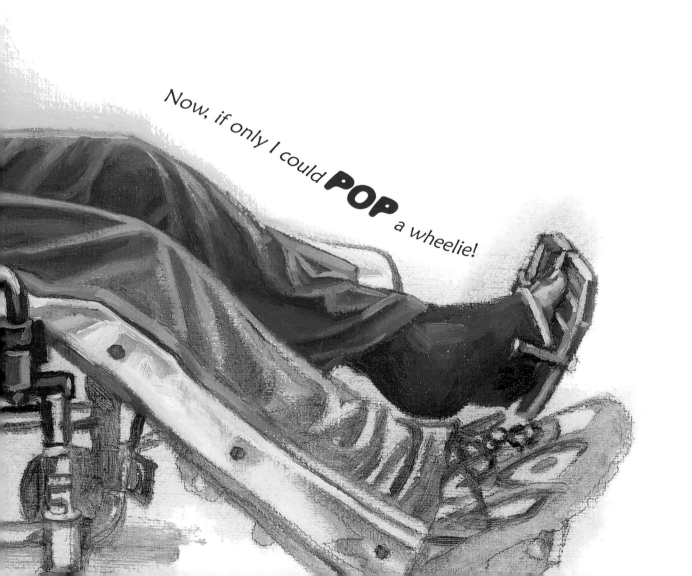

29

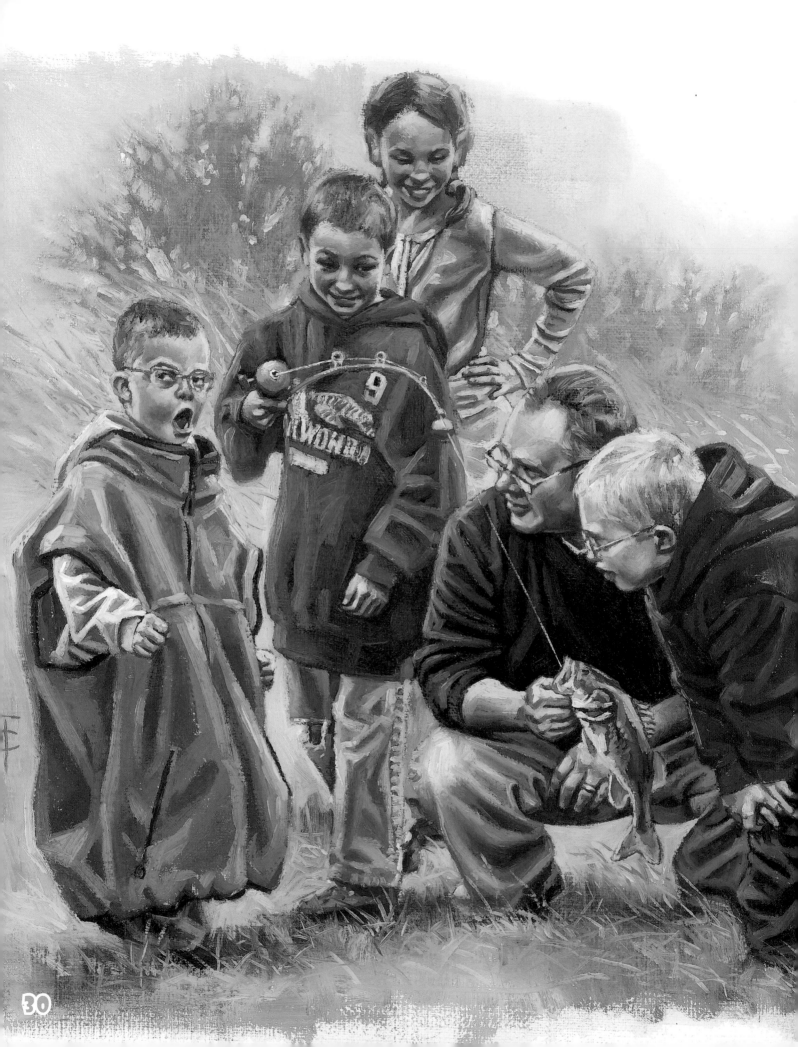

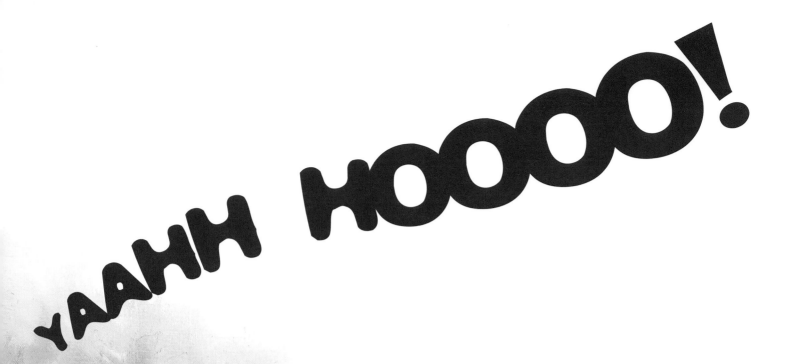

YAAHH HOOOO!

We also love to show our pals
we think they're great.

"When we catch a big one,"
says Lauren, "Louie *always*
cheers the **LOUDEST**."

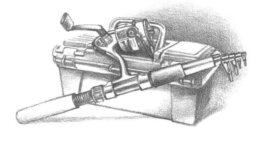

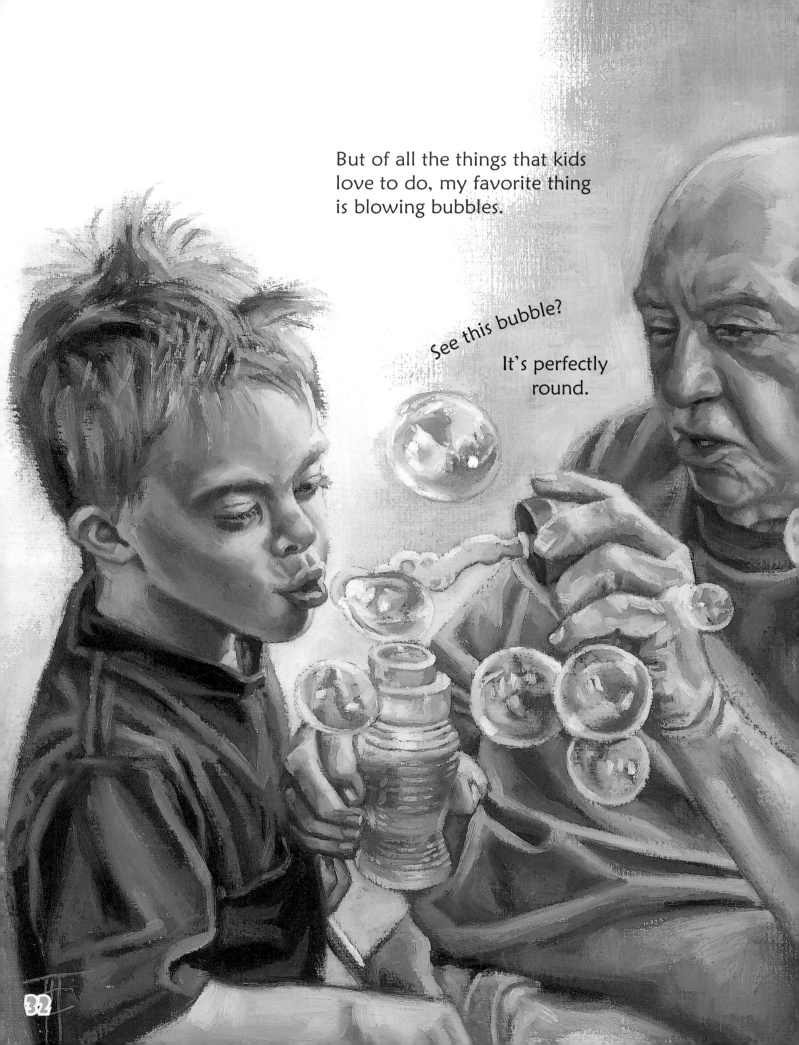

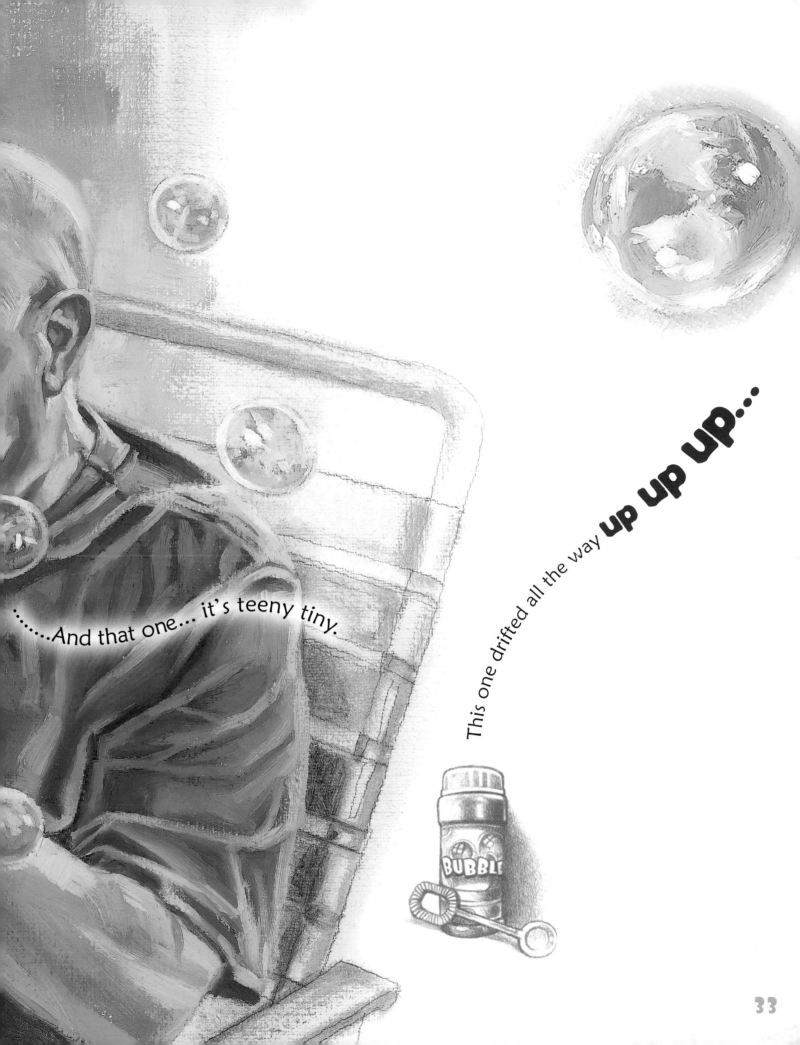

......And that one... it's teeny tiny.

This one drifted all the way **up up UP...**

BUBBLE

...into the clouds.

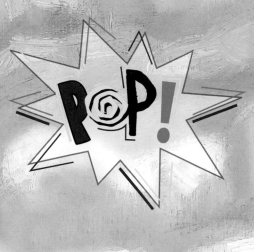

POP!

No two bubbles are exactly alike.

(That would be boring!)

But they're all bubbles. Right?
They're all made of
soap and water.
They all float in the air.

 It's the same with you and me.
No two kids are exactly alike.
But we're all kids. Right?

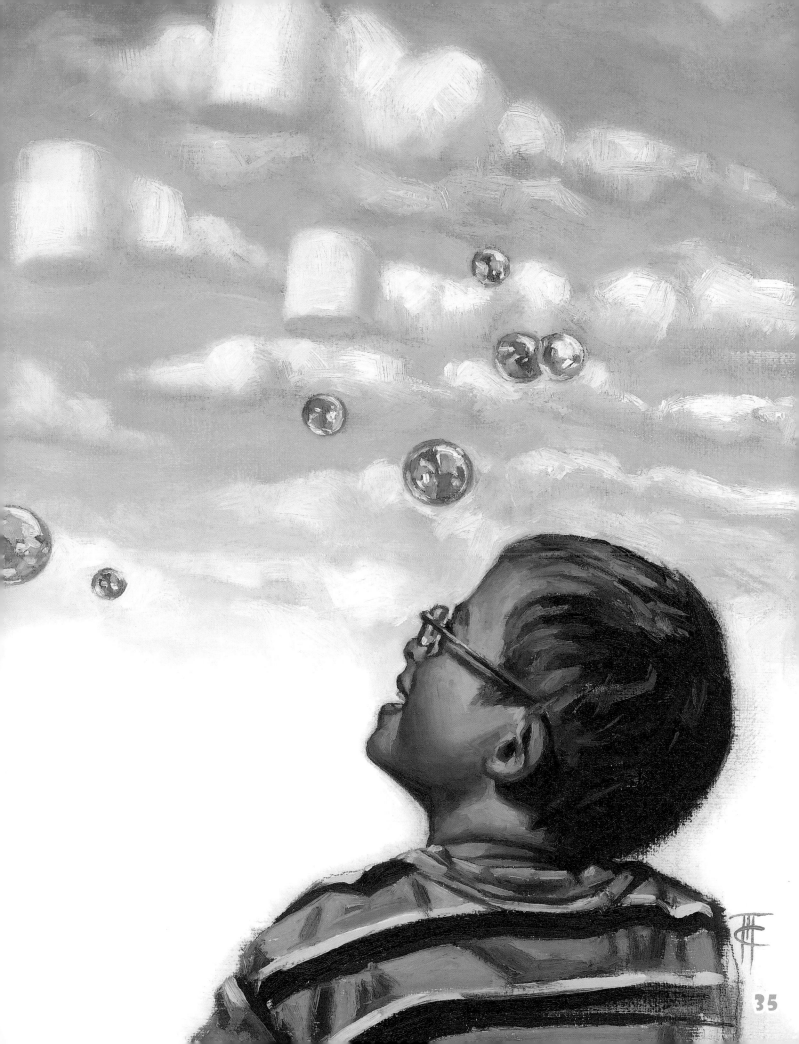

35

Of course we are!

And we love to use our imaginations.
So let's run and play in the Marshmallow Kingdom,
where the sun always shines and every meal's a picnic...
with marshmallows for dessert.

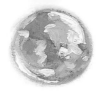

YUM!

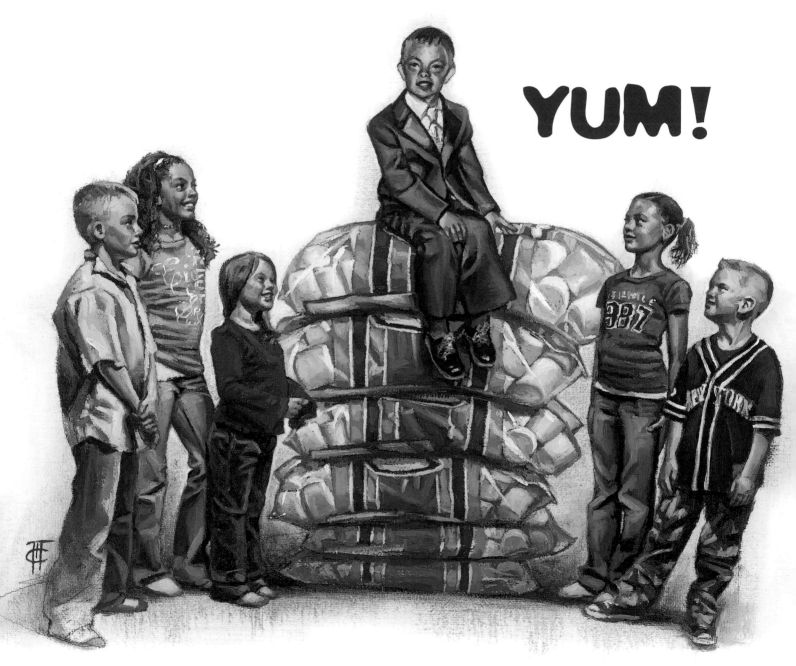

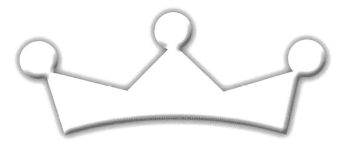

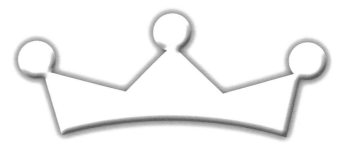

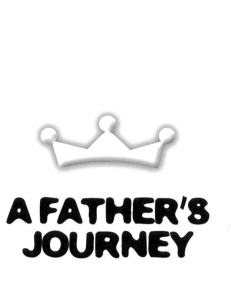

A FATHER'S JOURNEY

It's September 14, 2000. I'm in a room at Omaha's Bergan Mercy Hospital, and my mind is reeling. Moments earlier, several doctors have gathered in the room to tell my wife and me that our newborn son—our first child—was born with Down Syndrome. I don't know how exactly my life will change because of this. But from the moment I hear the news, I know that it will be unlike anything I could have anticipated.

During Jill's pregnancy, my dreams for this child became so vivid that, now, in this moment, I can't imagine their being thwarted. They run through my mind in a loop: I think about the soccer shoes. The small pair of Adidas soccer shoes that I ran out to buy when I knew we were having a boy—a boy who would (I just knew it), become an all-star athlete.

I think about high school, college, marriage, work—and all the plans I'd made in these areas for my son, sometimes even without realizing it. What am I supposed to do with all that? Where do people put their dreams when they know they won't come to pass?

One of the doctors in the room interrupts my thoughts. "I'm sorry," she says. "I know you wanted a happy, healthy child."

It's just one comment. From one doctor. And certainly, exceptional doctors were more the norm for us. Later, for instance, I would watch our primary doctor through the window of the neonatal intensive care unit. After a grueling shift, he visited the ICU to see Louie, rocking him tenderly in his arms.

The startling insensitivity of the comment thrusts me back into the here and now. And it's exactly what I need, because it activates the fight in me. In an instant, my spinning thoughts get clear:

Who is this person—a stranger—to come into this room and apologize for something as precious as human life? For something as precious as this human life—a boy with a name that's fit for a king: Louie the IV?

Suddenly, I fully apprehend: This isn't an occasion for shame. Or fear or sadness. This child, my firstborn son, is reason to celebrate.

Two years later, one evening just before Christmas, I learned just how much celebrating I could expect. For many years, my extended family had gathered at a favorite restaurant to share a holiday meal together. And every year, Joey, a young man whose family also frequented the restaurant, called on our table.

We looked forward to seeing Joey. And he looked forward to seeing us—not least because my dad gave him an annual Christmas envelope stuffed with $50. But ever since Louie had come into our lives, my connection with Joey ran deeper. Because Joey, in his 30s by then, also had Down Syndrome.

From the other side of the restaurant, he spotted me and Louie—and approached with his big smile. But when he saw Jill and my cousin Laura, his eyes widened: Both women were pregnant with their second children.

A businessman to the hilt, Joey managed his annual transaction with my father first, then turned his attention to family matters. "I'm going to do something for this family," he said, and gestured toward Jill and Laura. "Something to help you out."

Our interest piqued, we asked him to elaborate.

"I'm going to go home tonight," he said, "and I'm going to pray really hard—as hard as I ever prayed for anything—that all the rest of your children are born with Down Syndrome."

He smiled, rocking back on his heels—the better to bask in all the gratitude he was about to receive. Or so he thought. Instead, from one end of the table to the other, my family fell silent. Jill and I, on the other hand, could see the comment from Joey's perspective.

We exchanged a look—and burst into laughter. That put Joey in stitches. For a good while, the three of us were alone in our revelry. But eventually, the rest of the table came around to appreciating the humor of the situation.

From Joey's point of view, Down Syndrome was not a problem. It wasn't a fault or source of shame. Joey was immensely proud of who he was, and he viewed Down Syndrome as one thing that made him exceptional. He demonstrated this every time he introduced himself to someone new: "I'm Joey," he would say, "and I have Down Syndrome."

On hearing Joey's proclamation that night, the members of my family surely struggled to imagine how anyone could wish Down Syndrome on a child. Given all that it represented for Joey, however, I suspect that he couldn't imagine why anyone would not.

In the end, Joey's prayers didn't come true. But his message was clear: Often, when a child is born with a special need, the parents feel they must prepare for a lifetime of struggle. Joey was preparing us for something else entirely: A lifetime of joy.

I think of that night a lot. From time to time, a close friend will ask me if I think Louie "suffers" from Down Syndrome. I can't answer that question without talking about Joey. Like many people with Down Syndrome, he faced health problems throughout his life. In his case, a heart condition took his life too soon—at age 38.

You could safely say Joey suffered from that heart condition. Did he suffer from Down Syndrome? No way. Neither does Louie. My son doesn't really "do" suffering. It's just not his thing. But celebration? He does that like nobody's business.

I wrote this book about Louie for so many reasons. In part, I wanted another way to tell Louie how much I love him. But I was also inspired to write it because of what Louie tells the rest of us. Just by being himself, he reminds us that celebration is always possible, no matter how far our lives stray from what we had planned.

Less than a decade after that scene in the hospital, I found myself watching Louie, now 7, make his way up the green grass of a local soccer pitch. His form was impeccable. Even an elite athlete would have been impressed. Emblazoned across his jersey was a number "1". And on his feet: A pair of Adidas sneakers—the kind his dad had worn for years.

"Kid's looking great on that field," a fellow dad said, leaning in to congratulate me.

Squinting in the sun, I agreed. And I couldn't help but think about the day Louie was born. I wanted to go back in time—back to that hospital room where a new father was mourning the loss of his dreams.

I'd have told him that he hadn't lost anything—that he didn't need to retire his dreams, because they would come to pass after all. No, they wouldn't be exactly what he envisioned. But, in ways he couldn't understand yet, they'd be better: Richer, more interesting. Often, they'd be hilarious.

Like on this soccer field: My all-star athlete, the kid with the most exquisite form on the team, also happened to be moving in exquisitely slow-motion. Why? Just because. And if his dad were to pull him aside and explain that the object of this race was to come in first, he would have pitied his poor dad, a pretty cool guy who nonetheless just didn't get it.

With the other teammates on this soccer team for children with special needs, Louie played not to win—but to give and get love, to feel the sun on his face, and to relish the freedom of movement, step by (slow-motion) step.

In the 1987 prose poem, *Welcome to Holland*, Emily Perl Kingsley writes that having a baby is like planning a trip somewhere you've dreamed about for years. In Kingsley's poem, that place is Italy.

But from the start, she writes, the trip takes an unexpected turn. When your plane lands, you learn that you have arrived not in Italy, but—unbelievably—in Holland. What? Holland? You've never even considered Holland. You're confused. You want an explanation—but no one has one. You've landed in Holland and that's that.

There's nothing you can do but regroup and look around. Which is what you do, strolling the streets, visiting museums. You discover that Holland has tulips. Beautiful tulips. You discover windmills and Rembrandt. And in no time, to paraphrase Kingsley, you fall for Holland.

Louie, of course, is my "Holland." And for me, "Holland" is infinitely more glorious than anything I could have planned. "Holland" is a wonderland.

We recently discovered that, when our church congregation sings "Halleluiah," Louie thinks they're singing "Hah-lay-Louie."

That's what "Holland" is like.

Louie carries around a doll that, inexplicably, he named Jesus. As a result, Jill will catch herself at the grocery store saying things like: "No, Louie. You and Jesus cannot have that bag of marshmallows!"

That's "Holland," a place where everyday chores become sublime comedy.

It's a place where self-pity isn't welcome.

When Louie was diagnosed with type 1 diabetes, I was down in the dumps about it for weeks. Didn't my son have enough on his plate already? But one evening, Louie decided I'd done enough brooding. He called me over, and proceeded to sing a ditty, roughly to the tune of *La Cucaracha*: "I have di-a-BEE-teez. I have di-a-BEE-teez." This was accompanied by a jumpy little dance.

That's "Holland," a place where you sing and dance in the face of disease. To the tune of *La Cucaracha*.

When they're young, children have a flexible definition of "normal." The way that our 6-year-old daughter explains Louie to her friends bears that out. Even if he's acting out, Mia is matter-of-fact. "That's my brother Louie," she'll say, clomping up the stairs with her crew. "He has Down Syndrome, and sometimes he does silly things."

Her friends, all around age 6, take a few seconds to process the information. They nod—and then get on with their play. No big deal.

But in just a few years, those girls and boys will have received a stream of messages about what's normal and what is not. They'll have been encouraged to value sameness and to minimize or mask their differences. They'll have learned to reject anyone who doesn't conform to the rules set by the media or the restrictions defined by their neighborhoods, schools and other social and cultural groups of which they're a part.

This book is my way of sending an alternative message, one that encourages children to be themselves with confidence, eccentricities and all. My son Louie is pretty inimitable. But I've done my best to capture his spirit in this book because I know that, just by being himself, he challenges those social pressures to conform.

And he reinforces certain truths that very young children know instinctively: Until they're taught otherwise, they know that "normal" is overrated. That life is sweet in Holland. And that irrespective of race, gender, creed or special need, we people of the world are far more similar to each other than we are different.

—Lou Rotella III

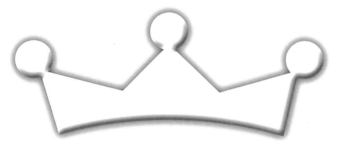

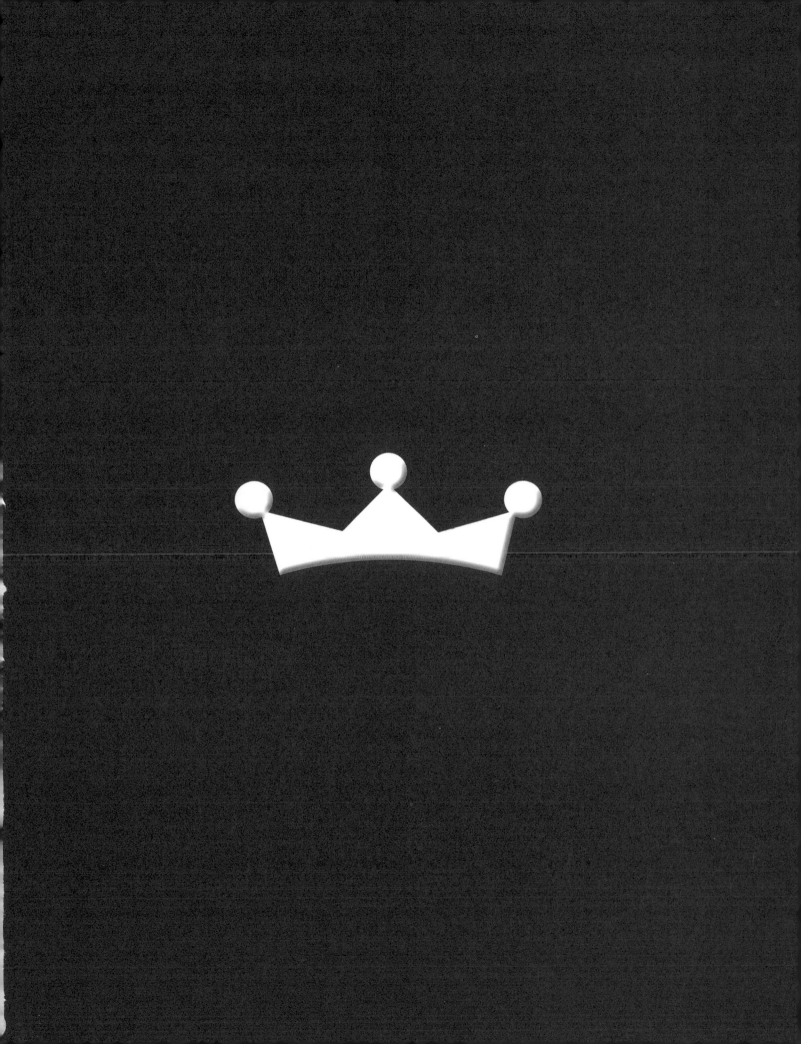